DIABETES

Can you Catch It?

By: Dana D. Carroll and Isaiah Smith

About the Authors

Isaiah was diagnosed at the mere age of two with type 1 diabetes. He has learned the struggles faced by a diabetic. It isn't always easy dealing with the fluctuations in blood sugar levels but he does the best he can. Dana is his grandmother and has watched him grow into a brave smart young man in his few years on this earth.

Copyright © 2022 Dana D. Carroll & Isaiah Smith

All rights reserved.

For

Bug

Diabetes

What is it?

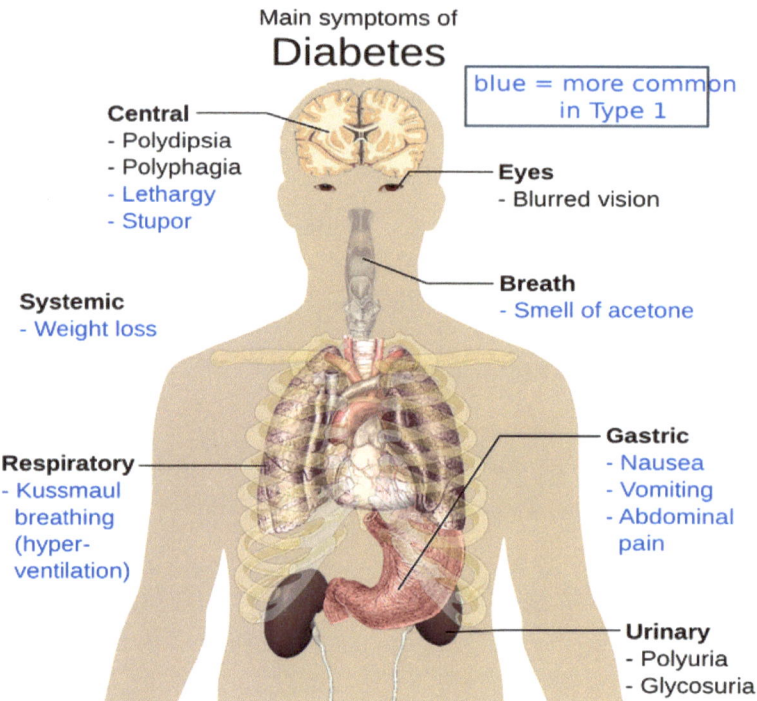

Diabetes is a group of diseases that affect how your body uses blood sugar known as glucose. Glucose is an important source of energy for the cells that makeup your muscles and tissues, it's also a source of fuel for your brain.

Can I catch It?

No diabetes is not contagious. The cause of diabetes is how glucose is processed in your body. Glucose comes from two main sources, food, and your liver. Your liver makes glucose. To counteract the glucose (sugar), a hormone from a gland called the pancreas secretes insulin. This insulin circulates letting the sugar enter the cells causing a drop in the blood glucose levels. As your blood sugar drops the secretion of insulin from your pancreas drops too, so a diabetic must check their blood sugar levels many times a day, by pricking their finger with a small needle called a Lancet. Some people have a pod that attaches to their skin called a Constant Glucose monitor that they can use to check blood sugar levels without pricking their finger.

Why do diabetics need to check their blood sugar?

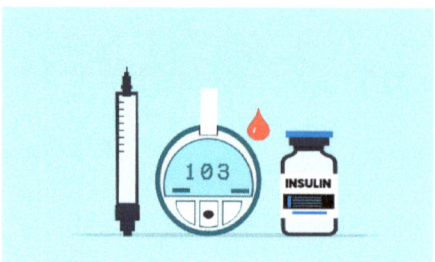

Diabetics have to check their blood sugar levels to be sure it doesn't get too high or too low. A test is performed at their doctor's office called an A1C this test shows how well their blood sugar is being controlled over a period of time. Numerous other blood tests are performed routinely, including checking cholesterol, blood pressure, kidney function and eye tests.

Highs and lows cause damage to their organs. It's very difficult to maintain a "normal" blood sugar level. Eating healthy and exercise and the proper amount of sleep can help, but there will still be times when blood sugar might be high or low. When glucose builds up in the bloodstream it's called hyperglycemia, a low is called hypoglycemia. There are signs and symptoms that alert them to a high blood sugar or a low blood sugar.

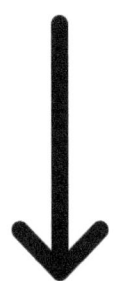

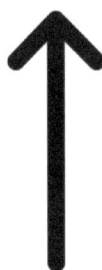

Signs to Look for

High blood sugar: Very thirsty, feeling hungry, Blurred vision, numbness, and tingling in feet, losing weight despite increased hunger, using the bathroom frequently, fruity breath, nausea, vomiting, flushed face, deep rapid breathing, dry ski skin and mouth, stomach pain, trouble focusing, tiredness.

Low Blood sugar: Headache, Hunger, Nervousness, Rapid heartbeat, Shakiness, Confusion, trouble focusing, tiredness, Weakness.

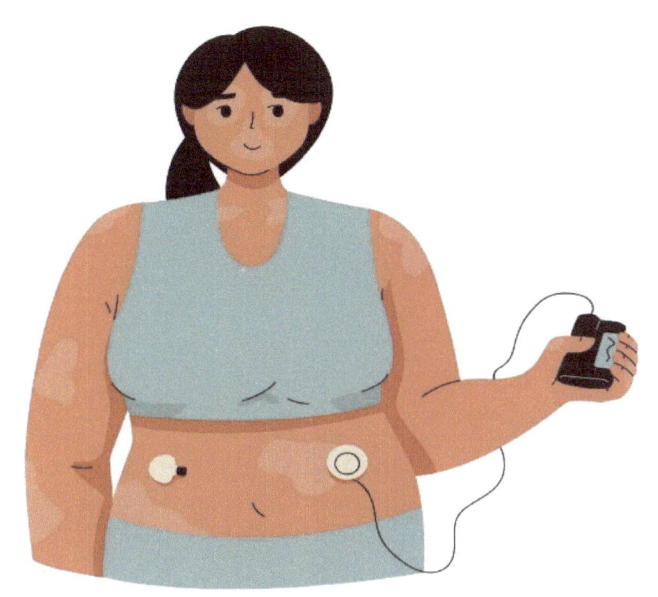

Diabetics might have to use a pump

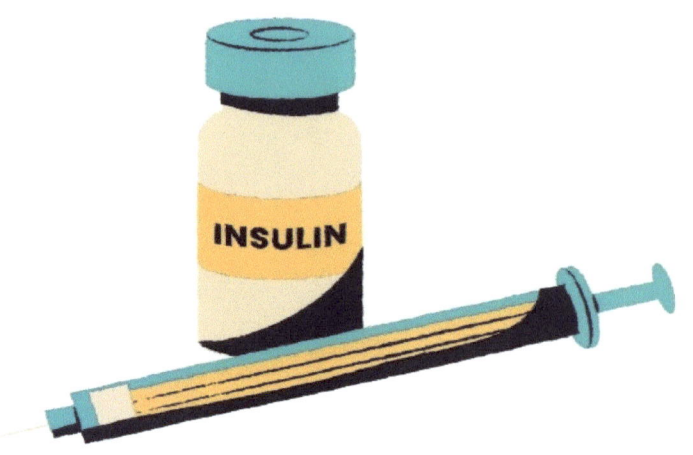

Diabetics often have to use insulin.

Diabetics have to be on alert because either a high or low could be detrimental. During heavy exercise they will need to take a break and have a snack to prevent a low blood sugar, and fluids to prevent overheating and dehydration. Staying healthy and well is the goal. If a diabetic person becomes sick they have to take extra care of themselves.

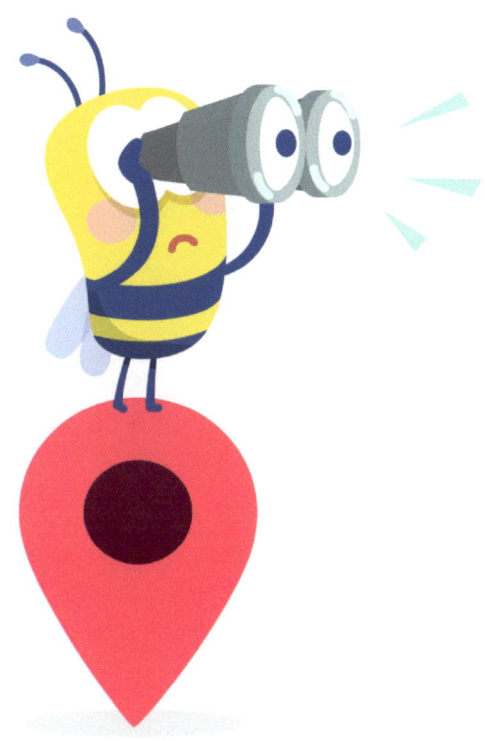

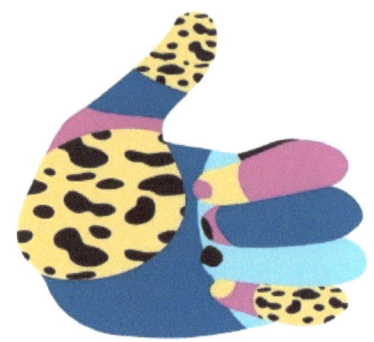

Can A diabetic person do the same things as everyone else?

Of course they can. The only difference is that they have to keep a check on their blood sugar levels. They are just as strong and capable as anyone else.

What can you eat if you have diabetes?

Diabetics can eat the same thing as everyone else, but they have to be cautious about how many carbohydrates are in their food. They have to count each carbohydrate and take insulin to cover the extra glucose. It's very important to eat healthy well- balanced meals and stay away from too many sugary, starchy of high trans-fat foods. A healthy diet includes fruit, vegetables, proteins, and water.

Can anyone become diabetic?

Yes. There are many Types of diabetes. If you become insulin resistant you may become a diabetic.

One type is Type 1. Type 1 diabetics are insulin dependent, but this type of diabetes is different. It is an autoimmune disease that makes the immune system attack the insulin making cells in your pancreas. It is a genetic disorder. There are 1.6 million Type 1 diabetics in the world. Type 1 can be triggered by a virus or cold, and genetics. The exact cause is unknown. Most are diagnosed as children. Their pancreas stop making any insulin after a certain amount of time.

Another type is Type 2. This is when your body doesn't use the insulin you produce properly or you don't produce enough insulin, you become insulin resistant.

So you will need insulin or other medications to help control blood sugar.

Type 2 develops over time and is seen in mostly adults but there are children and young adults that develop Type 2. This can be caused by a number of factors. Some risk factors are having a close family member that is diabetic, overweight, and physically inactive less than 3 times a week, age plays a role too. Anyone can be diabetic.

Diabetic people have to be cautious not only about food but also their physical and

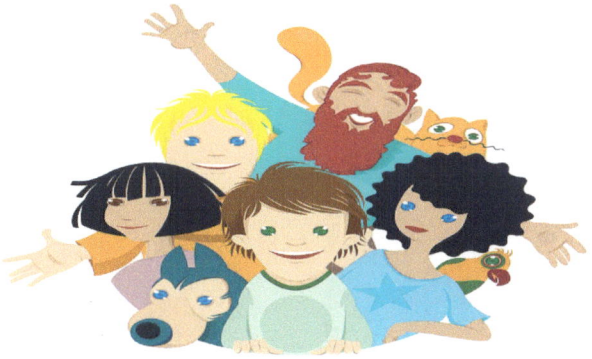

mental health. Sometimes diabetes can cause sadness, this is the time to take a break, listen to music, read, or just chill. There are other considerations too, like keeping a check on your feet, diabetics need to be careful, not only on the outside but inside too. Diabetes damages the organs in your body. So you will need to take extra care of yourself and control those blood sugar levels, watch what you eat and exercise.

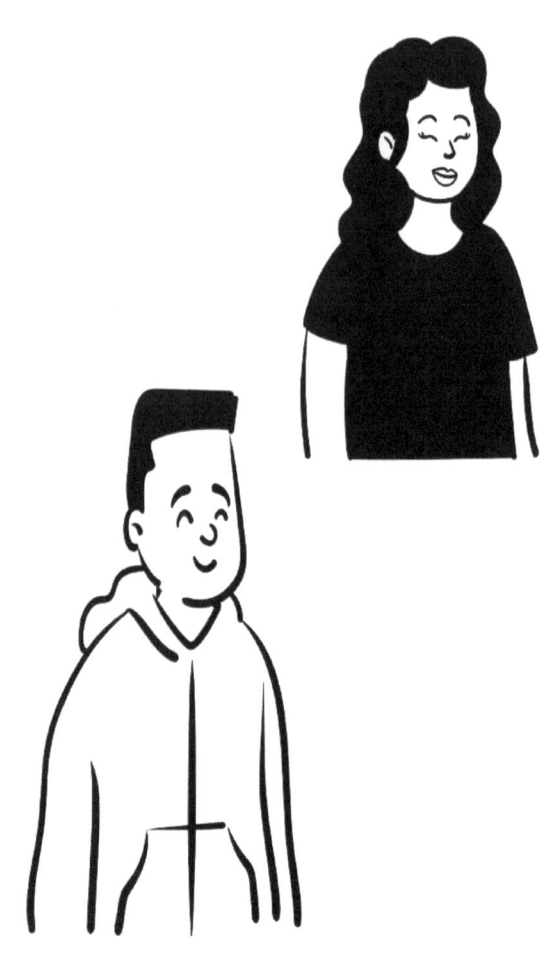

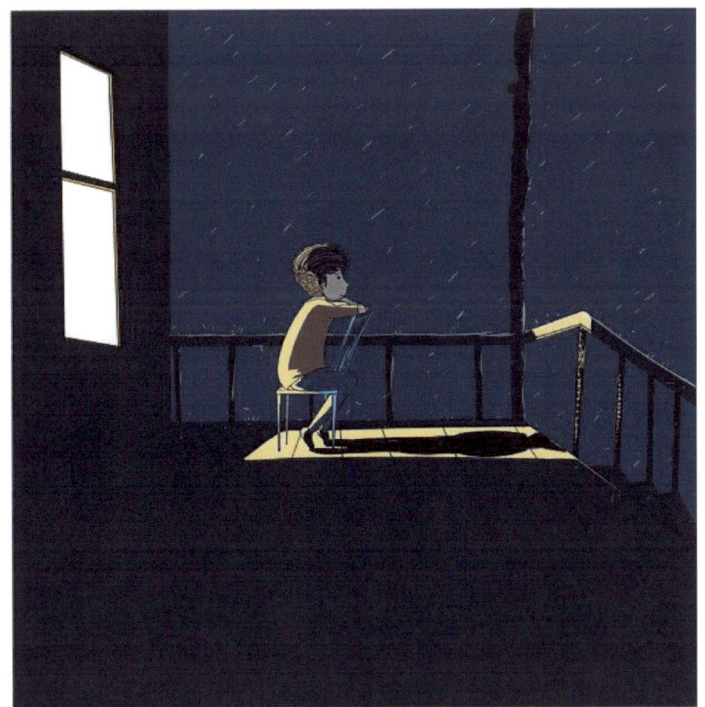

Most importantly remember to be the hero you are.

Is there a cure for diabetes?

Unfortunately there is not at this time. But medical technology has come a long way. There are many trials that are working on a cure, so there is hope.

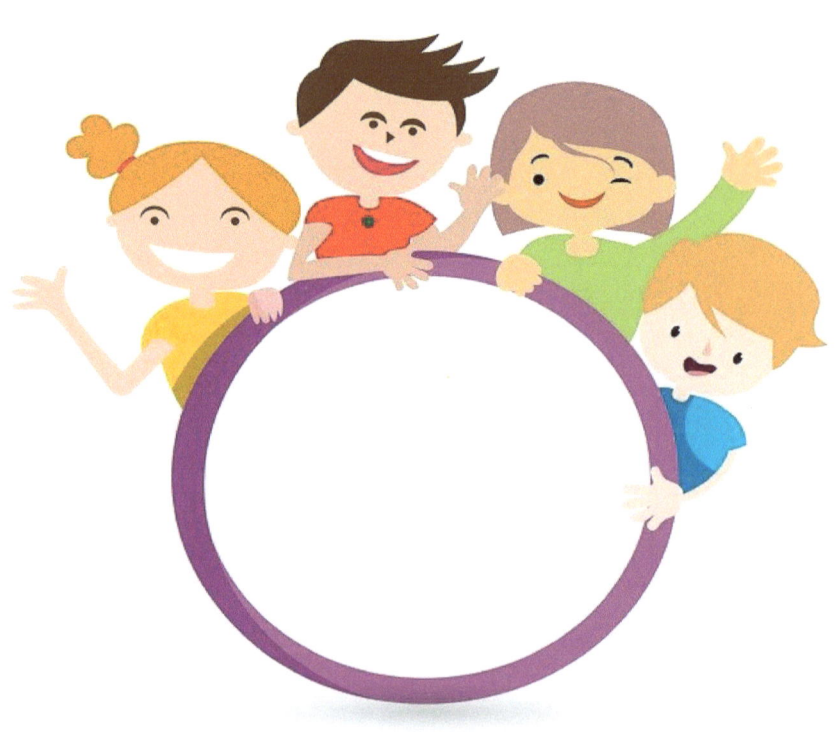

Hope For A Cure.

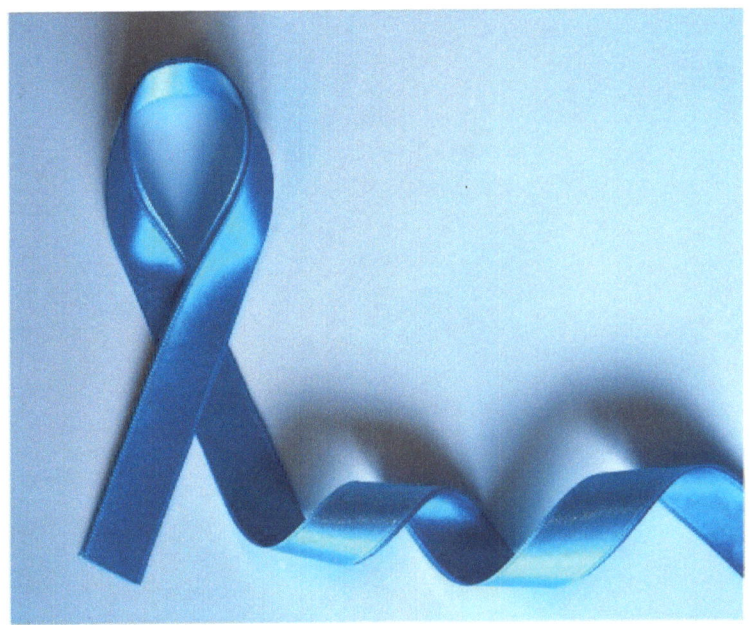

If anyone you know has diabetes be aware of signs and symptoms of a high or low blood sugar. You could save their life. Sometimes a drop or increase can happen so suddenly that person might need your immediate help. Call 911 and get help.

Check List for Diabetics:

Always have glucose meter

Always have insulin

Always have Glucose tablets

Always have protein bar

If you have a pump Always have extra pods

Always have Glucagon

Always have Emergency Contacts

Always be sure to alert friends/relatives/co-workers of possible emergency situations

Keep a watch on changing Blood Sugar Levels

Books by this Author

Diabetes Can You Catch It?

And Isaiah Smith

The Many Adventures of Newt

And Isaac Robinson

All Around the Town

And Micah Robinson

Kookaburra's Kooki Critter Alphabet

And Emma Kelley

The C word Cancer Stinks

Fiction Books by Dana D. Carroll

for ages 16 and above

Deception The Recombinant experiment

Deception The Final Phase Out of the Fire

The End

www.ingramcontent.com/pod-product-compliance
Lightning Source LLC
Chambersburg PA
CBHW040305220526

45473CB00002B/586